Dash Diet

Cookbook For Weight Loss With Action Plan And Easy Recipes

LELA GIBSON

LELA GIBSON

CONTENTS

Introduction

I want to thank you and congratulate you for buying the book, *"Dash Diet"*.

In an attempt to lose weight, we try almost any diet we can get our hands on. However, the sad thing is that most of these diets are just fad diets that don't offer long lasting results. It is important to point out that if you want to lose weight, you need to make a lifestyle change and not just adopting a diet for few days, losing a few pounds and gaining all that weight back after a while. This is why diets that are too restrictive are hard to adopt in the long run and this is where the DASH diet comes in.

The DASH diet is unlike any other diet because it focuses on lifestyle change rather than just losing a few pounds. Initially, the diet was started to help deal with high blood pressure; however, it is also quite effective in weight loss. The amazing thing is that it is not too restrictive and you can actually adopt it as a lifestyle. If you want to learn more about the DASH diet, what it entails and how you can use this diet to lose weight, this book will help you do just that.

In this book, you will learn more about the DASH diet, how it helps lower blood pressure and promotes weight loss, as well as some meal ideas, meal plans and recipes to get you started with the diet.

Thanks again for buying this book, I hope you enjoy it!

What Is The DASH Diet?

The DASH (Dietary Approaches to Stop Hypertension) diet is an eating planespecially recommended for those with pre-hypertension or hypertension (high blood pressure). This diet helps in lowering blood pressure by availing key nutrients such as magnesium, calcium, and potassium all of which are associated with lower blood pressure. The DASH diet is rich in vegetables, fruits, nonfat dairy or low fat. It also includes lean meats, poultry and fish, whole grains, beans and nuts.

While the DASH diet was initially developed to help lower blood pressure, it is now also considered quite effective in weight loss, promoting hearth health, lowering inflammation and cholesterol.

Let us learn more about how this diet can do all the above:

WeightLoss

To lose weight, you have to create a calorie deficit. The DASH diet does not stress on calorie reduction; however, it recommends consumption of whole grains, vegetables, fruits and lean meats. Whole grains, fruits and vegetables are high in fiber, which is quite filling but relatively lower in calories. Meat, poultry, and fish being protein take quite some time to be digested; hence, you feel fuller for longer. If you combine this and reduce your intake of processed sugars, sweets and unhealthy fats, you will create a caloric deficit without too much work, which will lead to weight loss.

The great thing is that you will not feel hungry even as you lose weight because all the foods you will be eating are quite filling.

LowersBlood Pressure

The DASH diet helps in lowering blood pressure due to its food composition. The DASH diet is rich in fiber, calcium, magnesium, and potassium; and has a low content of saturated fat and sodium. Adding more of these nutrients to your diet improves the electrolyte balance in your body thus allowing it to excrete the excess fluid that contributes to high blood pressure. These nutrients also reduce blood pressure by promoting the relaxation of blood vessels. Most people suffering from high blood pressure usually have these nutrients in deficiency so the DASH diet is quite effective at providing these nutrients; thus, lowering blood pressure.

Lower Cholesterol Levels

The DASH diet recommends intake of whole grains, which are high in fiber. Oats, brown rice, and whole-wheat products are excellent sources of fiber. Adequate fiber in your body has been shown to reduce cholesterol levels. Women should obtain 25 grams of fiber per day while men should aim for 38 grams.

Manages Insulin Resistance

The DASH is further favorable for those people with insulin resistance, pre-diabetes or diabetes as it helps in improving insulin sensitivity. The combination of nutrients and foods in the DASH diet may have an effect on various cellular targets that ultimately elevates changes in your body composition during weight loss thus effecting favorable impact on insulin action.

What To Eat And Avoid

As mentioned earlier, you should eat certain foods and avoid others while on the DASH diet. Let us look closely at the foods you can eat while on the DASH diet.

Foods To Eat

Vegetables: asparagus, artichokes, cabbage, mushrooms, bell peppers, cauliflower, beets, lettuce, onions, celery, broccoli, parsnips, Brussels sprouts, egg plants and corn

Fruit: apples, pineapples, blueberries, dates, kiwi fruit, papaya, mango, cherries, pears, apricots, plums, peaches, strawberries, honey dew, lemons, bananas, grape fruit, prunes, blackberries and tangerines

Non-fat or low fat dairy: Greek yogurt, low fat sour cream, feta cottage cheese, low fat buttermilk, mozzarella (part skim), chevre (goat cheese), soft parmesan cheese, low fat or fat free milk, trans fat free kefir, reduced-fat cheddar, Monterey jack

Lean proteins: fish fillets (plain), salmon, deli meat, turkey (skinless),chicken (ground, lean), shrimp, tofu, eggs, tempeh, beef: sirloin, round or flank and lean, pork

Whole grains: whole-wheat pasta, quinoa, amaranth, spelt, barley, wild rice, couscous, triticale, bulgur, kasha (buckwheat), millet, oats (old fashioned), and brown rice

Healthy snacks: bean-based spreads like black bean dip or hummus, raw veggie sticks and raw unsalted nuts, dried fruit popcorn, whole grain pretzels, whole grain crackers

Nuts and seeds: walnuts, sunflower seeds, pumpkin seeds, hazelnuts, cashews, almonds, nut butter

Beverages: sparkling water, herbal tea, low-sodium vegetable juice, 100% fruit juice, low-sodium broth

Foods To Avoid

The foods and drinks you should avoid while following the dash diet include foods high in salt and sugar as well as high fat snacks such as:

Canned soups

Sauces and gravies

White Bread and rolls

Cured meats and cold cuts

Processed Cheese

Salad dressings

Red meat that is not grass-fed

Pastries

Sugary beverages

Sodas

Salted nuts

Potato Chips

Cookies

Candy

With that information on the foods to eat and those to avoid, let us now learn how you can actually adopt the DASH diet.

DASH Diet Action Plan: How To Adopt The DASH Diet

You need to first begin by asking yourself what you will be eating, how to incorporate the DASH diet into your lifestyle, and what to do when you have to eat out among others things. The previous chapter mentioned the foods to eat and those to avoid; therefore, get rid of any food in the pantry or fridge that is not allowed on the DASH diet so that you don't give in to temptations.

Once you do this, stock up your kitchen with your favorite DASH diet allowed foods and snacks. To shop smart, create a shopping list for DASH allowed foods and carry it along with you when you go shopping. Also, use diet planning tools such as the daily DASH tracker and the weekly meal planner to plan your meals to avoid instances where it is time to eat and you don't have any clue as to what you should eat. Such scenarios are likely to lead to eating unhealthy foods, which will defeat the purpose of adopting the DASH diet.

Since the dash diet calls for a decrease in your sodium intake, below are ways you can use to reduce sodium intake:

- Learn the terms that indicate that a particular food is high in sodium such as broth, soy sauce, cured and pickled.

- Move away the saltshaker from where you are. "Out of sight, out of mind"

- Limit condiments such as pickles, catsup, mustard, and sauces that have salt-containing ingredients.

Sometimes, adopting the DASH diet can be quite difficult especially when you are used to eating unhealthy foods. In such cases, it is much better to slowly incorporate the allowed foods into your diet as you reduce the disallowed foods until you get used to the new foods because you stop eating the disallowed foods altogether. Below are effective ways of easily adopting the diet:

Slowly increase your intake of vegetables and fruits

The DASH diet plan recommends that you consume 4-5 servings each of vegetables and fruits each day for the standard 2,000-caloriediet. Therefore, if your plate is half full of simple carbohydrates and the other half is protein and vegetables, make an effort to ensure that vegetables are half of your plate with the other half being protein and your usual simple carbohydrates.Once you get used to eating more vegetables, you can then start eating complex carbohydrates.

To increase your fruit intake, instead of snacking on Potato chips, French Fries, a burger, some cookies, cake or candy, have a fruit instead. You can opt to have some berries, a slice of pineapple, mango, watermelon, or apple. You can also make a delicious smoothie with all your favorite fruits. The good thing is that the fruit will give you that sweetness that you may be looking for in high sugar snacks while still providing other essential nutrients. In addition, fruits are more filling and you are likely not to overeat on fruits as compared to cookies, which are very easy to overeat without providing any essential nutrients.

Incorporate a few servings of low-fat dairy products every day

Rather than completely avoiding high fat dairy products, incorporate the low-fat variety. Low-fat yogurt with some fresh fruit makes a great snack or breakfast option. You can also add milk and yogurt to homemade smoothies or even snack on an ounce of cheese with whole grain crackers or nuts. If you don't eat dairy products you instead can have non-dairy alternatives with minimal added sugar.

Switch starchy and sugary snacks for whole foods

The DASH diet eating plan doesn't leave you with much room in your calorie budget for traditional processed snacks such as cookies and chips. You need to select snacks that incorporate whole foods such as whole grains, low-fat dairy, nuts, fruits, and vegetables. Below are some friendly DASH-friendly picks:

1 cup edamame in the pod

1/4 cup unsalted nuts

Whole grain crackers with 1 ounce cheese

Veggies with hummus or bean dip

Plain, low-fat yogurt topped with fresh fruit

Celery sticks, banana or apple with 1 tablespoon nut butter

3- 4 cups air-popped popcorn

Limit red meat – choose poultry, fish, and beans instead

While red meat is allowed on the DASH diet, you should limit its consumption. Further, ensure that you eat grass-fed meat and not grain fed meat, which is high in saturated fat and omega 6 both of which contribute to obesity, high blood pressure and heart disease and promote inflammation. This is why red meat that isn't grass fed is not allowed on the DASH diet.

The DASH diet recommends 6 ounces of lean protein each day with fish, beans, and chicken being among the top choices. Most Americans eat plenty of poultry but most of them struggle with incorporating more beans and seafood into their diet. Load up on your legume intake by substituting canned, low-sodium beans for animal proteins in pasta dishes, chili, tacos, entrée salads, and hearty soups.

In addition, to the above steps, in the following chapter, I will provide you with more tips on getting started with DASH diet as well as being successful.

DASH Diet Tips

As you start the DASH diet, below are some tips that can help you. These include:

Embrace meal planning

It is difficult to follow any diet without a bit of planning. The same applies to the DASH diet too. You need to know the type of foods you have in your pantry and freezer. A previous chapter has provided you with this information comprehensively. This way, you can know what to buy and cook. Many people find it beneficial to prepare meals for the week. You don't have to cook everything if you don't want to. However, you do have to make a conscious effort to have the foods you need available whenever you need them.

Buy in bulk

There are many foods allowed in the DASH diet that you can buy in bulk. Things such as brown rice, whole-wheat pasta, meat and even canned foods can be purchased and stored for later. However, don't just shop without a plan. Instead, make a list of all the items you need to purchase.

Also, it is important to check expiry dates especially when you're buying in bulk. It would be unfortunate to buy a lot of food only to find out that they will be expiring within a short time. Do your homework and make wise purchasing decisions. You should also have a storage system that allows you to use items with shorter expiry dates first. You don't want to waste any food.

Buy in-season produce

Of course, you have to eat fruits and vegetables when you're on the DASH diet. This does not mean that you insist on eating only certain fruits and vegetables. Expand your horizon and look for options that are easier to find and cheaper. You can do this by purchasing in-season produce. Buy both ripe and unripe fruits to stretch the use of the produce. Also, look into drying and freezing fruits such as berries. This way, you can still eat such fruits even in the off-season months.

Cook your meals at home

You need to cook most of your meals at home if you want total control over what you're eating. When you cook at home, you get to choose which food items you want to use. For example, instead of using processed foods, you can select whole foods. You can make it a goal to do batch cooking. This way, you'll have a lot of food to freeze for later. If you do batch cooking, you should remember to freeze the food in individual containers. This will make your work easier as you'll only need to remove the container you plan on using during mealtime.

Another thing to note is that cooking at home is definitely less expensive than constantly eating out. It is also an opportunity to bond with your family.

Take a moment to read food labels

Don't just pick up food items and place them in your shopping cart without first reading the labels. Labels contain nutritional facts that will guide you when it comes to selecting the right foods

You should be particularly interested in the amount of sodium in such foods. Foods that are low in sodium have less than 140mg per serving and products that claim to be very low in sodium should have less than 35mg per serving.

Also, make it a point to look for reduced sodium products and low fat products. These alternatives make it possible to select items that are healthier in the long run.

Alternate your sources of protein

You do not have to eat meat each day. You can embrace other sources of protein. Foods such as beans, lentils, peanut butter and peas are great sources of protein.

It would also be wise to eat more vegetables and fruits than proteins. You should select low calorie foods and foods that are not high in carbs. For example, you should make it a habit to eat more berries than high carb fruits such as bananas. This will be good for your weight, as you won't have to worry about calories adding up.

Beware that your choices add up

The choices you make are not made in isolation. At the end of the day, you'll have to account for all the appetizers, snacks, meals and desserts you eat. When you select what to eat and drink, you have to make healthier choices that will be better for you each day. If you want to select drinks, you can choose water, diet soda, club soda, coffee, tea or fruit juice. However, you have to remember to take the above drinks in moderation. For instance, drinking too much fruit juice would be counterproductive as such juices are often high in carbs. Drinking too much caffeine would also work against your health.

You should also be careful when selecting appetizers, soups and salads. Try to go for healthier choices. Your salads, for example, should contain plenty of green vegetables. You also need to check the salad dressing to ensure it is in line with the DASH diet. Avoid eating foods with extra meats, cheese or eggs. You can enjoy such things but you don't need to overdo it.

Another area that deserves your caution has to do with baked foods. You should make it a point to halve things such as butter and sugar whenever you're baking. Use whole grains and natural sweeteners instead of processed foods and artificial sweeteners whenever you can. This way, you'll still be able to enjoy plenty of recipes while you're on the dash diet.

The following chapter will provide you with some ideas for DASH diet breakfasts, lunch, dinner and dessert as well as a 4-day meal plan.

DASH Diet Meal Ideas

Adopting a new diet is quite challenging especially when you are not quite sure where to start. In this chapter, I will give you some easy tips on how to change your meals and make the DASH diet friendly:

Breakfast

- When you are having scrambled eggs or omelet be sure to add chopped vegetables (broccoli, tomatoes, spinach, mushrooms)

- Instead of water, prepare oatmeal with low fat milk then top with a few nuts and sliced fruits

- Have a cappuccino or latte made with low fat or fat-free milk

- Pour yourself a bowl of whole-grain cereal along with low fat milk then add berries, banana slices, or dried fruit

- Make a breakfast parfait: layer granola or whole grain cereal, fruit and low fat yogurt in a tall glass

- Spread nut butter on whole grain toast then top with raisins, pear, apple and sliced banana

- Top ½ whole grain English muffin with a slice of low fat cheese and tomato sauce then place under the broiler for the cheese to melt

- For a quick smoothie, blend a banana or frozen fruit, 100% fruit juice and low fat yogurt

Lunch

- Instead of soda or any other soft drinks, drink low fat or fat free milk, sparkled water

- To prepare soup, use low fat milk instead of cream and water

- Top salads with pineapple chunks, seeds, crunchy nuts, dried fruits, grapes, mandarin orange sections and diced apples

- Enjoy broth based bean, lentil or vegetable soup or head for the salad bar

- Add extra vegetables such as grated carrots, mixed greens, peppers, and tomatoes to your sandwich

- Add extra frozen or fresh vegetables to canned or homemade soups

Dinner

- Begin your meal with a large green salad

- Grill or roast vegetables such as cauliflower, carrots, eggplant, mushrooms, zucchini, onions, and peppers and drizzle with balsamic vinegar

- Make one-pot meals with whole grains such as quinoa, buckwheat, bulgur, brown rice and barley; and peas or beans

- Stir-fry colorful vegetables then bite size pieces of tofu, shrimp, pork, or chicken with a bit of your desired stir-fry sauce

Dessert

- Fruit has always been natures perfect dessert – just sink your teeth into something that is juicy, sweet and in season:

- Try baked bananas, pears, or apples with a scoop of low-fat frozen yogurt

- Top low fat vanilla yoghurt with in-season, ripe berries and a sprinkle of sliced almonds

- For a tasty BBQ treat, grill fruit skewers over medium-hot coals

- Using berries, grapes, bananas, melon chunks and pineapple, create fruit kabobs

Below is a four-day DASH diet meal plan that you can adopt:

DASH Diet Meal Plan

Day 1

Breakfast:½ cup (75 grams) of blueberries, 1 cup (90 grams) of oatmeal with 1 cup (240 ml) of skim milk

Snack:1 medium apple

Lunch: mayonnaise andtuna sandwich made with 3 ounces (80g) of canned tuna, 1.5 cups (113g) green salad, 2 slices of whole grain bread, 1 tablespoon of mayonnaise, 1 cup (248g) vegetable soup

Snack: 1 medium banana

Dinner: 3 ounces (85g) of lean chicken breast cooked with ½ cup (75g) carrots, ½ cup (75g) broccoli and 1 teaspoon of vegetable oil. Served with 1 cup (190g) brown rice

Day 2

Breakfast: Scrambled eggs with vegetables, ½ cup (120 ml) fresh orange juice

Snack: 1 medium orange

Lunch: 3 ounces (85g) of lean turkey, ½ (38g) cup of green salad, 1.5 ounces (45g) low-fat cheese, ½ cup (38g) cherry tomatoes, 2 slices of whole wheat bread and 1 teaspoon of unsalted butter

Snack: 4 whole grain crackers and 1.5 ounces (45g) of cottage cheese

Dinner: 1 cup (200g) of mashed potatoes, ½ cup (75g) of broccoli, ½ cup (75g) green peas and 6 ounces (170g) of cod fillet

Day 3

Breakfast: 2 slices of turkey bacon, ½ cup (38g) of cherry tomatoes, 1 teaspoon of unsalted butter, 2 slices of whole wheat toast with a cup of tea made with skim milk

Snack: 1 cup Greek yogurt

Lunch: ½ cup (38g) of salad greens, 1 tablespoon of low-fat mayonnaise, ½ cup (38g) of cherry tomatoes, 1.5 ounces (45g) of low fat cheese and 2 slices of whole wheat toast

Snack: 1 cup of fruit salad

Dinner: Whole-wheat pasta and meatballs made with 4 ounces (115g) of turkey meatballs and 1 cup of pasta and ½ cup (75g) of green peas

Day 4

Breakfast: 1 cup (90g) oatmeal with ½ cup (75g) of blueberries, 1 cup (240 ml) of skim milk

Snack: 1 medium pear

Lunch: chicken salad made with 2 cups (150g) of green salad, 3 ounces (85g) of lean chicken breast, ½ cup (75g) of cherry tomatoes, 1 tablespoon of mayonnaise, ½ tablespoon of seeds

Snacks: 1 handful nuts

Dinner: 3 ounces of roast beef with ½ cup (75g) of broccoli and 1 cup (150g) of boiled potatoes.

I bet you are quite excited to get started with the diet. In the following chapter, we will look at some DASH diet recipes that you can try out.

Are you enjoying this book? Leave a review on Amazon!

DASH Diet Recipes

Breakfast Recipes
Vegetable Omelet

Yields: 4 servings

Ingredients

1/2 cup shredded reduced-fat sharp cheddar cheese (2 ounces)

1/8 teaspoon cayenne pepper

1/8 teaspoon salt

2 cups fresh baby spinach leaves or torn fresh spinach

8 eggs

2 tablespoons Italian (flat-leaf) parsley

Nonstick cooking spray

1 recipe Red Pepper Relish (see recipe at the end of whole recipe)

Directions

Use cooking spray to coat the inside of a nonstick skillet (10-inch) with flared sides. Heat the coatedskillet over medium heat.

Combine the cayenne pepper, salt, parsley, and eggs in a large bowl. Use a wire whisk or a rotary beater to beat ingredients until frothy.

Pour the frothy mixture to the prepared skillet then immediately begin to stir the eggs continuously but gently with a plastic or wooden spatulauntil it looks like cooked egg surrounded by liquid egg. Stop stirring and cook until the egg is set but shiny for 30-60 more seconds.

Sprinkle the egg with cheese once it is set but still shiny. Top with ¼ cup of the red pepper relish and 1 cup of the spinach.

Lift one side of omelet and fold partially over filling using a spatula. Arrange the rest of the spinach on a warm platter then transfer the omelet to the platter.

Top with the remaining relish

Red pepper relish recipe

Combine ¼ teaspoon of black pepper, 1 tablespoon of cider vinegar, 2 tablespoons of finely chopped onion or green onion and 2/3 cup of chopped red sweet pepper

Tasty frittata

Yields: 4 servings

Ingredients

1 cup sweet cornfrozen

1 cup grape tomatoes, cut in half

1 cup sliced pepper strips

1 tablespoon diced fresh basil (or 1 teaspoon dry basil)

2 tablespoons canola oil

4 ounces shredded Jack/colby cheese or other cheese blend

6 eggs

1/4 cup sliced onion

Directions

Stir the eggs and basil in a small bowl.

Add the canola oil to a non-stick frying pan over medium heat. Once the oil is hot, add frozen sweet corn, onion, and pepper strips. (If desired, you may substitute a frozen mixture of onions and pepper strips).

Sauté the mixture for 3 minutes while stirring and turning over.Add the tomatoes and continue stirring and turning over. Cook for 5 more minutes until the onions become translucent.

Pour the egg-basil mixture onto the vegetables. Use a spatula to separate slightly in the interior or to lift the edges in order to allow the eggs to fall to the bottom of the mixture while the frittata cooks.

Top with cheese once the egg mixture has thickened all the way through then brown for 2-3 minutes under broiler.

Tip: ensure that you use a pan with metal handle since plastic is will most likely melt under the broiler. You could for instance try using an All-Clad pan.

Turkey Breakfast Sausage

Serves: 8

Ingredients

1/4 teaspoon ginger, ground

1/2 teaspoon pepper

1/2 teaspoon rubbed sage

3/4 teaspoon salt

1 pound lean turkey, ground

Directions

In a large bowl, crumble your turkey and then add in pepper, sage, ginger and salt. Shape the turkey into 8 two-inch patties.

Cook over medium heat in a non-stick skillet that is coated with cooking spray, for 4-6 minutes on each side.

When done, the juices should run clear with a thermometer reading of 165 degrees Celsius.

Healthy Breakfast Salad

Serves: 1-2

Ingredients

Oil for frying the eggs

2 eggs

¼ teaspoon sea salt

1 tablespoon olive oil

¼ cup of pine nuts, toasted

1 small handful of parsley, roughly chopped

1 small handful of fresh basil, chopped

1 not too ripe avocado, diced

1 red pepper, diced

2 large handfuls of cherry tomatoes, halved

½ English cucumber, thickly sliced

Directions

In a large bowl, combine together olive oil, pine nuts, all veggies and salt and toss well.

Then over medium heat, heat a cast iron or a skillet and add a splash of oil. Once the pan is hot, add eggs to the pan. Consider adding a little splash of water to facilitate to eggs get cooked.

Finally, remove the eggs from the skillet and serve with the salad.

Grain-Free Almond Bread

Serves 3

Ingredients

1/2 teaspoon baking soda

2 cups almond flour, blanched

1/2 cup almond butter or coconut oil, melted

1/2 teaspoon sea salt

1/4 cup flax seed meal

1 tablespoon raw apple cider vinegar

3 -4 eggs

Directions

Preheat an oven to 350 degrees F.

Beat the eggs and vinegar in a mixing bowl, and then add in coconut oil and butter. Then whisk the mixture together until well blended.

Combine baking soda, salt, flax seed meal and almond flour in a separate bowl. Using a fork, mix until the mixture is well distributed. To this mixture, add flour mixture and combine to until well incorporated.

At this point, press the mixture into an 8 or 9-inch square baking pan and bake until golden brown, in about 30-35 minutes.

Cool down the bread for 15 minutes and then cut into 9 squares. If necessary, cut the squares horizontally, and drizzle with almond butter or coconut oil.

Lunch Recipes

Tuna Sandwich

Yields: 1 serving

Ingredients

1 5 ounce can low sodium tuna packed in water, drained

1/3 cup cherry tomatoes, sliced

1/3 cup fresh arugula or other leafy greens

1/4 cup reduced fat whipped cream cheese

2 green onions, sliced

2 slices hearty multigrain bread

2 tablespoons extra-virgin olive oil

2 tablespoons fresh parsley, chopped

2 tablespoons freshly squeezed lemon juice

Black pepper

Directions

Add the tuna to a medium sized bowl and set aside. Add the green onion, pepper, parsley, lemon juice and oil in a separate bowl and whisk to combine. Pour 2/3 of your oil mixture into the bowl of tuna and mix well.

Coat both sides of the bread lightly with the remaining oil using a pastry brush or spoon. Grill the coated bread over medium high heat in a non-stick skillet until it is golden on both sides. Toss the remaining oil mixture with the arugula.

To assemble the tuna sandwiches: on each side of the grilled bread spread 2 tablespoons of cream cheese. Add ½ of the tuna mixture to each of the slices followed by ½ of the greens and finally top up with ½ of the cherry tomatoes.

Pork with Apples

Yields: 4 servings

Ingredients

1 1/2 tablespoons balsamic vinegar

1 1/2 tablespoons fresh rosemary, chopped

1 cup low-sodium chicken broth

1 pound pork tenderloin, trimmed of all visible fat

1 tablespoon olive oil

2 cups chopped apple

2 cups chopped onion

Freshly ground black pepper, to taste

Directions

Preheat your oven to 450 degrees F.

Use cooking spray to coat a baking pan lightly.

Heat olive oil in a large skillet over high heat then add the pork. Sprinkle pork with black pepper and cook for about 3 minutes until the tenderloin has browned on all sides then remove skillet from heat.

Transfer the pork to the prepared pan, put it in the oven, and roast the pork until a food thermometer indicates 165 degrees F (medium) for around 15 minutes.

Meanwhile, add the rosemary, apple, and onion to the skillet. Sauté for around 3 to 5 minutes over medium heat until the apples and onions are soft.

Stir in the vinegar and broth then increase heat and boil for about 5 minutes until the sauce has reduced.

To serve: place the roasted pork on a large platter then slice on the diagonal and place on 4 warmed plates. Top the pork with the apple-onion sauce and serve immediately

Stuffed Bell Peppers

Serves 4

Ingredients

Salad or veggie of choice

Avocado or pre-made guacamole

Spices of choice

2 raw eggs

1 zucchini, chopped

1 fresh diced tomato

2 garlic cloves, chopped, or garlic powder

1 onion, chopped

1 pound beef or turkey, ground

2 bell peppers

Directions

First preheat your oven to 375 degrees F.

In a large skillet, brown the meat and then add garlic and onions. Cook the mixture for 4 minutes and then add in zucchini. Cook for 3 additional minutes.

Once done, remove the skillet from heat and now add in eggs, spices and tomatoes. Combine well to blend.

Cut off the tops from the peppers, and reserve them. Then scoop the seeds and now spoon the meat mixture into them. Use the meat that remains to make meat balls.

At this point, bake the ingredients in the oven for 30-40 minutes inside the glass baking dish. Once the peppers turn slightly brown, remove from heat.

To serve, top with the avocado or guacamole and the salad.

Chicken and Lettuce Wraps

Serves 1-2

Ingredients

1 small head of lettuce (4-5 leaves)

1 pinch Salt and pepper

1/4 cup 0% Greek yogurt

1 chicken breast, boneless, skinless; cooked and diced

1 tablespoon red onion, finely chopped

1/4 cup cucumber, diced

1/4 cup red bell pepper, diced

1 small green apple, diced, unpeeled

Directions

Mix together the above ingredients in a bowl apart from the lettuce. Let it chill for about 1 hour.

Then put the chicken mixture into each lettuce leaf and then roll into the cylinders before serving.

Enjoy!

Dinner Recipes

Tuna and spinach sandwiches

Yields: 4 servings

Ingredients

2 ribs of celery, diced

2 tablespoons of olive oil

Juice of 1 lemon

8 slices 100% whole wheat sandwich bread

1/2 medium cucumber, peeled, seeded, and diced

1/2 teaspoon of dill weed

1 cup of fresh baby spinach

1/2 teaspoon of salt-free seasoning blend

1/2 small red onion, peeled and diced (about 1/4 cup)

1/4 teaspoon of freshly ground black pepper

1 6.4-ounce pouch of light tuna packed in water

Directions

Combine the dill weed, celery, onion, cucumber, and tuna. Drizzle tuna mixture with lemon juice and olive oil then stir. Season with the freshly ground black pepper and salt-free seasoning blend

Make the sandwich with ¼ cup of the baby spinach leaves and ½ cup of the tuna salad. Press down to compact the spinach and the tuna

Note: This recipe yields 2 cups of tuna that you can keep in the fridge for up to 3 days in order to make more meals.

Roasted Squash with Wild Rice

Yields: 6 servings

Ingredients

1 cup diced onion

1 small orange, peeled and segmented

1/4 cup chopped walnuts

1/4 teaspoon thyme

2 teaspoons canola oil, divided

1 cup fresh cranberries

4 cups cooked wild rice

1/2 tablespoon chopped Italian parsley

4 cups diced winter squash, peeled and cut into half-inch pieces

Black pepper to taste

Directions

Preheat your oven to 400 degrees F.

Add the squash to a roasting pan and toss with 1 teaspoon of oil.

Roast until brown for 40 minutes. Brown the onions in a hot sauté pan with the rest of the oil. Add the cranberries to the browned onions and sauté for 1 minute.

Add the rest of the ingredients and sauté until heated thoroughly for around 4 to 5 minutes

Serve.

Mushroom Chili

Yields: 4 servings

Ingredients

½ cup of sliced ripe olives

1 (19 ounces) can of white kidney beans(rinsed and drained)

8 ounces (about 2-1/2 cups) of sliced shiitake mushrooms

1 (14-1/2 ounces) can stewed tomatoes

1 ½ pounds (about 7-1/2 cups) of white button mushrooms, sliced

1 teaspoonof ground cumin

2 tablespoons of chili powder

1 tablespoon of minced garlic

1 cup of chopped onion

2 tablespoons of vegetable oil

Directions
Heat oil in a large sauce pan until hot then add the garlic and onion. Cook for about 5 minutes stirring frequently until the onions become tender.

Stir in the cumin and chili powder and cook for about 30 seconds until fragrant

Add the shiitake and white button mushrooms and cook for 6 to 8 minutes stirring occasionally until the mushrooms become crisp tender.

Add ½ cup of water, olives, beans, and stewed tomatoes. Simmer for about 10 minutes to blend flavors.

Serve with tortillas; garnished with shredded cheddar cheese, diced fresh tomatoes and shredded lettuce if desired.

Spring Green Kale Salad

Serves: 2

Ingredients

1/2 cup raw pistachios

3 scallions, sliced

2 cup asparagus, sliced 1-inch pieces

3 kiwi, thinly sliced

2 large pear, thinly sliced

1 large bunch of kale, chopped

For dressing

Sea salt

1 tablespoon maple syrup

Zest of one lemon

3 tablespoons fresh lemon juice

3 tablespoons raw hemp oil

Directions

In a large bowl, pour in the kales that has been washed and torn into bite-sizes.

Add in the dressing and massage into the chopped kales until it is well coated and soft.

Now add in the other ingredients and toss to combine. Serve and enjoy.

Desserts

Oatmeal Walnut Cookies

Yields: 49 Cookies

Ingredients

1/2 cup chopped walnuts

1 cup bittersweet or semisweet chocolate chips

1 tablespoon vanilla extract

1 large egg white

1 large egg

2/3 cup maple syrup

4 tablespoons of cold unsalted butter, sliced into pieces

1/2 cup tahini (see Ingredient note)

1/2 teaspoon of salt

1/2 teaspoon baking soda

1 teaspoon of ground cinnamon

1/2 cup of whole-wheat pastry flour

1/2 cup all-purpose flour

2 cups of rolled oats

Directions

Position racks in the lower and upper thirds of the oven and preheat oven to 350 degrees F.

Line 2 baking sheets with silpat silicone liners or parchment paper.

Whisk the baking soda, rolled oats, salt, cinnamon, whole-wheat flour, and all-purpose flour in a medium bowl

Beat the tahini and butter in a large bowl using an electric mixer until the 2 ingredients are well mixed and form a paste.

Add the maple syrup and continue beating until ingredients are well-combined (note that the resulting mixture will be somewhat grainy)

Beat in the large egg followed by the egg white and finally the vanilla. Using a wooden spoon, stir in the oat mixture until just moistened. Stir in the walnuts and chocolate chips.

Roll a tablespoon of the batter into a ball with damp hands then place it on the prepared baking sheet. Flatten the batter ball slightly ensuring that the sides do not crack. Do this with the rest of the batter leaving a 2-inch space among the flattened balls.

Bake the cookies for about 16 minutes until golden brown switching the pans top to bottom and back to front halfway through.

Leave the cookies to cool on the pan for 2 minutes then move them to a wire rack to cool completely. Before baking another batch, leave the pans to cool for a few minutes. Store the cookies in an airtight container for up to 2 days. Freeze cookies for longer storage

Ingredient note: Tahini is a paste made from grinding sesame seeds. You can get it in some supermarkets and natural foods stores.

Chocolate Banana Cake

Yields: 18 Servings

Ingredients

2 cups all-purpose flour

1 large egg

1 teaspoon vanilla extract

1/2 cup Splenda Brown Sugar Blend

1/2 teaspoon baking soda

1 large ripe banana, mashed (1/2 cup)

1 egg white

1/2 cup semisweet dark chocolate chips

1/4 cup unsweetened cocoa powder

1 tablespoon lemon juice

3/4 cup soy milk

1/4 cup canola oil

Directions

Preheat your oven to 350°F.

Use nonstick spray to coat an 11 by 7 inch brownie pan.

In a large bowl, whisk together the baking soda, cocoa, brown sugar blend and flour

Whisk together the vanilla, lemon juice, egg white, egg, oil, soy milk and bananas in another bowl.

Make a hole in the middle of the flour mixture, and then pour in the chocolate chips and soy milk mixture.

Stir the ingredients together using a wooden spoon until well mixed then pour then spoon the batter into your prepared brownie pan

Bake for about 25 minutes until when you press the centre of the cake lightly with fingertips it springs back.

Hotcakes with Mixed Berries

Serves 10

Ingredients

Organic oil or grass-fed butter

Warmed frozen berries

1/4 teaspoon pure liquid stevia

1/2 teaspoon baking soda

1/2 teaspoon cinnamon, ground

2 teaspoons pure vanilla extract

4 whole eggs

8 ounce raw pecan pieces

Directions

Pulse your pecans in a food processor or blender to obtain a fine pecan meal. Then pour the pecans into a large mixing bowl and then whisk together along with stevia, baking soda, cinnamon, vanilla and eggs.

In a pan, warm some butter or oil and then ladle about 2 tablespoons of batter in the pan.

Cook the pancake until light and fluffy on both sides. Your hotcakes should fluff up when cooking.

Then in the microwave or pot, warm the frozen berries and then ladle them onto your hotcakes and serve.

Blueberry Cheesecake

Serves 8

Ingredients

2 cups blueberries

2 cups non-fat milk

2 packages sugar free cheesecake pudding mix

1 container fat free whipped dessert topping

Directions

Mix the pudding mix with milk and then pour half the mixture into a glass.

Place half the blueberries onto the pudding and press into the pudding.

Mix half the whipped topping with the remaining pudding mixture and pour this mixture on top of the blueberries and the spread to smooth.

Spread the remaining whipped cream on top then sprinkle the remaining blueberries on top. Refrigerate for 2 hours or more until set.

Snacks

Banana Smoothie

Yields: 2 servings

Ingredients

2 cups vanilla soy milk

1 banana, peeled

2 packets Splenda

1/2 avocado, pitted and peeled

1/4 cup unsweetened cocoa powder

Directions

Add all the ingredients to the blender and process until smooth then serve immediately

Chili Chai Hot Chocolate

Serves 2

Ingredients

1 tablespoon coconut oil

1 red chili

1 teaspoon cinnamon powder

1 teaspoon cardamom powder

1 inch of root ginger sliced

2 tablespoons organic cacao powder

1 tablespoon almond butter

450ml coconut or almond milk

Directions

Slice the ginger and then add it into a sauce pan. Add in the oil, spices, almond butter, cacao and milk.

Then simmer the mixture for about 5-10 minutes and then pour into a food processor or blender. Process the contents on high speed to obtain a smooth frothy substance.

To serve, sprinkle with cinnamon and enjoy.

Blueberry Muffins

Yields: 12 muffins

Ingredients

1 cup low-fat milk

1 egg

1-1/2 cupswhole-wheat flour

1/2 teaspoon baking powder

1/2 teaspoon salt

1/2 cup old-fashioned whole oatmeal (raw)

1/3 cup maple syrup

1/4 teaspoon baking soda

1/4 cup oil

2/3 cup frozen blueberries

Directions

Preheat your oven to 350 degrees F.

Use cooking spray to coat the inside of a muffin tin. Mix the dry ingredients (salt, baking soda, baking powder, oatmeal, and flour) in a bowl.

In another bowl mix all the other ingredients (egg, oil, milk, maple syrup). Pour the mixed wet ingredients onto the mixed dry ingredients then mix. Add the blueberries and gently stir; the resulting batter should be lumpy.

Scoop the batter into the muffin tins and bake until the muffins brown on the edges for around 20 minutes.

Serve warm or cool on a wire rack and store in the refrigerator in an airtight container.

Soft-Boiled Egg

Serves 1

Ingredients

Pepper

Salt

1 large organic egg

Directions

Fill a small deep-sized saucepan with 4 inches water then bring it to a boil and then reduce the heat to simmer the water.

Next, lower in the egg and set the timer to 6 minutes. Once ready, remove the egg and run it under cold tap for 15 second

Then place it into an egg cup and slice off the top third. To serve, season with salt and pepper and enjoy.

Vanilla Pumpkin Seed Clusters

Serves: 30

Ingredients

Water, boiled

2 teaspoon coconut sugar

2 teaspoon honey

1 teaspoon vanilla extract

½ cup pumpkin seeds

Directions

Preheat an oven to 150 degrees Celsius, and then combine vanilla, coconut sugar and honey in a small bowl.

Stir together to produce thick paste, and then add in a drop of boiled water; to create runny syrup. Pour the pumpkin seeds and stir to evenly coat the seeds.

Dollop a teaspoon of pumpkin seeds onto a baking sheet, and repeat the operation until it's all used up.

Cook the contents for about 15-20 minutes to brown the seeds. Then remove from the oven and cool for some time.

After cooling, press the clusters together to ensure they don't fall apart. Serve once cool and dry.

Healthy Dark Chocolate

Yields 100g of dark chocolate

Ingredients

Seeds of 1 vanilla bean

2½ tablespoon cocoa powder

1½ tablespoon maple syrup

3½ tablespoons cocoa butter

Directions

Over low heat, melt cocoa butter in a small sauce pan and then stir in vanilla bean seeds, cocoa powder and maple syrup. Whisk the mixture until smooth.

Temper the chocolate using a candy thermometer. Heat to 120 degrees F and then cool into the fridge at 79 degrees F. Keep for 10-15 minutes and ensure to stir every 5 minutes.

Remove from the fridge and heat at a constant temperature of 87 degrees F.

Finally pour into the mold, cool and then store the chocolate under refrigeration.

I need your help..

Thank you again for buying this book!

I hope this book was able to help you to understand the DASH diet, why it is effective in lowering high blood pressure, how you can lose weight once you adopt this diet, what to eat, and the foods to avoid, how you can easily adopt the diet as well as some tasty recipes that you can try out. The next step is to take action NOW and adopt the diet because you can never know how great it is until you try it out.

Finally, if you enjoyed this book, then I'd like to ask you for a favor, would you be kind enough to leave a review for this book on Amazon? It'd be greatly appreciated!

I want to reach as many people as I can with this book, and more reviews will help me accomplish that!

If you have any questions or problems, please contact us: hello@freedomdestination.com

Thank you and good luck!

Preview Of '20 Easy And Fast Diet Tips For Losing Weight'

Before we start learning about the strategies you can use to lose weight, let's start by highlighting some of the benefits that will come as a result of shedding those extra pounds just to give you extra motivation to want to do something NOW.

Why You Need To Lose Weight

Healthy weight loss has over one hundred benefits; these include emotional and physical benefits. I will dedicate this section to discussing the health benefits that many people (and weight loss/health books) do not pay enough attention to.

1: You Avoid Pre-Diabetes or Type 2 Diabetes

Pre-diabetes/high blood glucose is a condition that develops when the blood sugar levels in your blood move past normal ranges but not enough to qualify as diabetes. When your body stops consistently producing insulin sufficient to meet your body's needs, or the amount produced does not work properly, type 2 diabetes is likely to develop. Being pre-diabetic places you at a very high risk of developing type 2 diabetes.

Being obese or overweight is a proven leading risk factor for type 2 diabetes because carrying excess weight typically makes it hard for cells to respond to insulin, and since the additional fat acts as an insulating layer, it makes it more difficult for the sugar to enter the cells, which results in more circulating blood sugar levels.

Nonetheless, if you are already a pre-diabetic, you can prevent the progression to diabetes by shedding some weight (to reduce the insulating layer on cells so that they respond more to insulin) and trying to maintain a healthy weight.

2: You Keep Your Heart Healthy

When it comes to heart disease, some of the key risk factors are high cholesterol and high blood pressure. Research shows that:

1. Excessive accumulation of body fat makes your body release particular chemicals that occur naturally into the bloodstream, which increases blood pressure, and

2. Being overweight makes the liver produce too much amounts of Low density Lipoprotein (LDL) also called cholesterol. LDL tends to be sticky and gathers in the walls of blood vessels, which causes the narrowing of arteries, a condition called atherosclerosis, which increases your risk of strokes and heart attack.

When you lose weight, your blood pressure often reduces and the liver naturally reduces the amount of LDL it produces.

Royal Adelaide Hospital conducted a research on cardiovascular improvements with respect to a special weight loss program. Their results showed a decrease of cholesterol by 12%, a 10% decrease of LDL, a 5% decrease in diastolic blood pressure, and an 8% decrease in systolic blood pressure.

3: Improved Sleep (and Possible Treatment of Sleep Apnea)

One of the most prominent benefits of losing weight is improved sleep. When you gain excess weight, you gather more soft tissues in the neck; this intensifies the incidence of snoring.

NOTE: Snoring is a result of constricted airways, which obstructs air movement.

Snoring can be a symptom of sleep apnea, a possible life-threatening condition characterized by obstruction of breathing that requires the victim to wake up frequently from sleep to resume breathing.

As a victim of sleep apnea, you rarely remember anything about the episodes of waking many times a night to breathe but even so, this sleep and oxygen deprivation could easily lead to a weak immune system, high blood pressure, heart disease, memory problems, and sexual dysfunction.

When you lose weight, you reduce the amount of fatty tissue in the back of your throat, decrease snoring and the likelihood of the worsening of your health- as aforementioned. You encourage better sleep quality and reduce the risk of developing sleep apnea.

4: Better Joints (Mobile and Pain-Free)

Osteoarthritis (OA) is one of the most common joint disorders. It causes the tissues that protect the joints (cartilage and bone) to wear away. Consequently, the joints become tender and swollen, thus making movement very painful.

When you are overweight, you add to the load placed on the joints that bear the weight such as hips and knees.

NOTE: When you walk, you exert a force of approximately 3-6 times your entire body weight across the knee (read more on this page (check the discussion section) or here), so adding about 10 kg of weight does increase the force on the knees, which is equal to carrying 30-60 kgs^2 extra.

Therefore, a loss of merely 5% of your body weight could reduce the amount of stress placed on the knees, lower back, and hips, and reduce the pain (remember that losing 5kgs is equal to relieving a force of 15-30kgs^2 on the knees). According to doctors, a 10% loss of bodyweight has presented a 28% improvement in knee osteoarthritis symptoms.

5: Improved Fertility

There is epidemiological evidence that proves being obese has negative effects on reproduction. There has not been clarity in the mechanisms underlying the relationship between infertility and obesity but research studies suggest that excess body can lead to a serious offset in the metabolism of sex hormones that produce menstrual disruption and consequently, subfertility.

Moreover, when you are pregnant and overweight, you a more likely to miscarry and (or) develop other medical complications, and in particular, gestational diabetes, pregnancy induced hypertension, thromboembolism, and preeclampsia. There are reports to show that deliveries in obese women show increased rates of labor induction, caesarian section, and problematic labor caused by increased size of the unborn baby.

Additionally, experts report that a baby of an overweight woman is more likely to require more medical attention (admission to neonatal intensive care) and develop congenital defects such as cardiac and neural tube problems.

Moreover, obese individuals are more likely to experience birth related injuries and the likelihood of giving birth to babies with large birth weights, which puts them at risk of birth trauma and a possibility of childhood and probably lifelong obesity. Reducing weight in this case could help you and your baby avoid all these health problems.

Emotional Weight Loss Benefits

The negativity usually around overweight people affects your self-esteem and confidence. Naturally, when you are carrying some excess weight, you will worry about how other people see you and become overly anxious in particular situations. This affects many aspects of your life including your job interactions and performance, school, and your life at home (in the neighborhood).

Losing weight will help you gain confidence and increase your self-worth and self-love; losing weight normally makes you cheerful and as a result, your relationships with other people improve. Most of your fears and anxieties related to being overweight disappear and in general, you live a better life.

Once you regain your confidence, you feel in control. This becomes the status quo once you become comfortable with your new weight. Once you lose the weight, you are more comfortable when making food related decisions.

You also feel and become more honest when you interact with others and can better articulate your thoughts and feelings. You will no longer hold back since you are more self-possessed about your appearance and health.

Now that you know some of the benefits you stand to gain from losing weight, let us discuss the various effortless ways to lose weight.

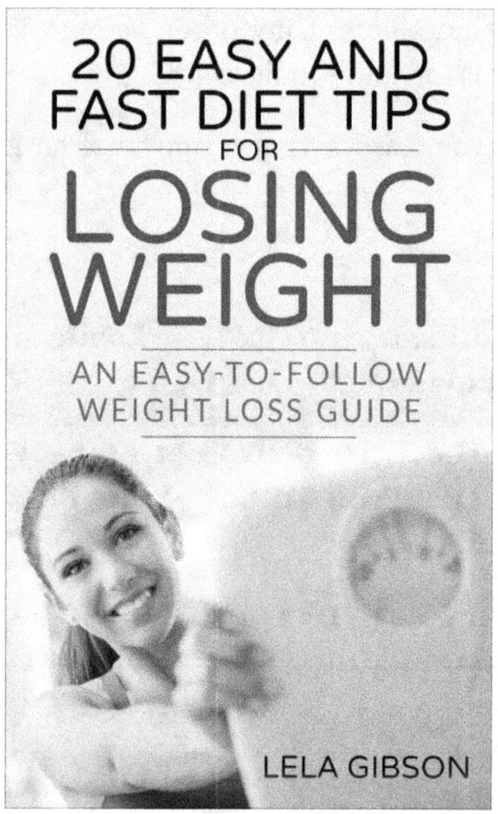

Check out the rest of 20 Easy And Fast Diet Tips For Losing Weight on Amazon, go to: http://amzn.to/2mNtPEg

Check Out My Other Books

Below you'll find some of my other popular books that are popular on Amazon and Kindle as well.

Alternatively, you can visit my author page on Amazon to see other work done by me.

20 Easy And Fast Diet Tips For Losing Weight — An Easy-To-Follow Weight Loss Guide

Belly Diet: The Zero Belly Diet Step-By-Step Guide Which Will Help You To Lose Your Belly And Enjoy Your Flat Belly

Anti-Inflammatory Diet Guide — The Guide To Reduce Inflammation And Live A Healthy Life Without Pain

Clean Eating: Cookbook And Guide To Restore Your Body's Natural Balance And Eat Healthy

Negative Calorie Diet: Cookbook & Guide Which Help You To Burn Body Fat, Lose Weight And Live Healthy

Smart Fat: Cookbook With Fat Meals Which Help You To Lose Weight, Get Healthy And Improve Brain Function